30-DAY FOOD GLOW WORKBOOK

Companion to the 30-Day
Food-Based Skin Health Book

STEPHANIE WILLIAMS, MBA

Entrepreneur | Strategic Business Consultant |
Real Estate Investor and Mentor

BOOKED & BRANDED
PUBLISHING

COPYRIGHT

Published by Booked and Branded Publishing
www.bookedandbrandedpublishing.com

ISBN: 978-1-969369-27-8

Disclaimer: This book is for informational purposes only and is not a substitute for professional medical advice, diagnosis, or treatment. Always consult a qualified health provider before making changes to your diet or supplements.

📩 hello@bookedandbrandedpublishing.com

DEDICATION

To everyone choosing nourishment over noise. May your plate, your skin, and your life glow — from the inside out.

TABLE OF CONTENTS

TABLE OF CONTENTS

TABLE OF CONTENTS

TABLE OF CONTENTS

WELCOME

Welcome + How to Use This Workbook

This workbook is your practical partner to the 30-Day Food-Based Skin Health Book. Use it to track your food, hydration, and habits as you move through the 30-day challenge.

- Read the chapters in the book.
- Complete the worksheets here.
- Check in with yourself weekly to celebrate wins and note progress.

This is your space. Make it personal.

CHAPTER 1

Your Glow Goals

Prompt: In 30 days, I want my skin to…

My top 3 skin goals are:

1. ______________________________

2. ______________________________

3. ______________________________

CHAPTER 2

My Current Skin & Nutrition Habits (Self-Audit)

Check what applies to you right now:

- ☐ I drink at least 70 oz of water daily
- ☐ I eat vegetables with every meal
- ☐ I eat processed sugar daily
- ☐ I eat omega-3 rich foods (salmon, walnuts, chia)
- ☐ I eat probiotic foods (yogurt, kimchi, sauerkraut)
- ☐ I drink alcohol more than 2x per week
- ☐ I get 7–8 hours of sleep
- ☐ I manage stress daily (journaling, walking, meditation)

Reflection: What habits need improvement first?

CHAPTER 3

Hydration Tracker (Week 1)

Daily Goal: ______ oz

Days	Cups/oz Drank	Notes (skin, energy)
Monday		
Tuesday		
Wednesday		
Thursday		
Friday		
Saturday		
Sunday		

CHAPTER 4

Vitamin C & A Focus (Week 1)

Daily Log:

Omega-3s I ate today: ______

Leafy greens I ate today: ______

Nuts/Seeds/Avocado: ______

Reflection: Did my skin feel more hydrated or balanced?

CHAPTER 5

Probiotics & Minerals (Week 3)

Track probiotics + mineral-rich foods:

Probiotic food today: ________________________

Zinc-rich food today: ________________________

Iron-rich food today: ________________________

How did my digestion feel today?

____

____

CHAPTER 6

Antioxidants & Collagen (Week 4)

List your daily glow foods:

Antioxidants: ______________________________

Collagen/Protein: ______________________________

Vitamin C booster: ______________________________

Reflection: Do I notice firmer skin or less dullness?

____

____

CHAPTER 7

Meal Planning Worksheet

Weekly Food Plan

Days	Breakfast	Lunch	Dinner	Snacks
Monday				
Tuesday				
Wednesday				
Thursday				
Friday				
Saturday				
Sunday				

CHAPTER 8

Glow Grocery List

Staples for Radiance

- Citrus (lemons, oranges, kiwi)
- Leafy greens (spinach, kale, collards)
- Salmon or other omega-3 sources
- Avocado, nuts, olive oil
- Probiotics (yogurt, kimchi, kefir)
- Bone broth
- Green tea, blueberries, dark chocolate

Blank space to add your own:

CHAPTER 9

Skin Troubleshooting Log

Issue: (acne, dryness, dark circles, dullness)

What I ate yesterday: _______

Hydration: _______

Stress level: _______

Sleep hours: _______

Possible trigger: _______

Adjustment for tomorrow: _______

CHAPTER 10

Recipe Reflection Page

Recipe tried: _______

Rating (1–10): _______

Substitutions I used: _______

Would I make this again? [ ] Yes [ ] No

CHAPTER 11

30-Day Challenge Habit Tracker

Stay organized and thorough when screening tenants for your rental properties.

Days	Hydrati on	Vitamin C	Healthy Fats	Probio tics	Antiox idants	Glow Notes
1st						
2nd						
3rd						
4th						
5th						
...30th						

CHAPTER 12

Skin Progress Check-In (Before/After)

Day 1 Reflection:

How does my skin look today?

Energy level: _______

Mood: _______

Day 30 Reflection:

My biggest change is: _______

Energy level: _______

Mood: _______

(Optional: add progress photos here.)

CHAPTER 13

My Top 5 Glow Foods

Journal prompt:

Which 5 foods gave me the most visible results?

1. ____________________

2. ____________________

3. ____________________

4. ____________________

5. ____________________

CHAPTER 14

My Long-Term Glow Plan

Questions:

Which daily habit will I keep forever?

____

____

How will I balance food + topical glow care (Glow Up Skincare)?

____

____

What new skin goal will I set for 90 days?

____

____

CHAPTER 15

Motivation Page (Quote Wall)

Quotes to keep you glowing:

- "Glowing skin is always in."
- "Every bite is skincare."
- "Consistency is the new magic."

Space to add your own mantra:

FINAL REFLECTION

My skin feels:

The most surprising thing I learned:

My next step is:

WORK WITH ME

You've invested in your glow — now let's build your next transformation.

Visit www.bookedandbrandedpublishing.com to explore

- Ghostwriting + Publishing Services
- Strategic Business Consulting
- Branding + Customer Experience Strategy

Email: hello@bookedandbrandedpublishing.com

ABOUT THE AUTHOR

Stephanie Williams, MBA, Strategic Business Consultant, author, and builder of beauty, brains, and business.

Stephanie Williams is the founder of Booked and Branded Publishing and the creator of the Glow Up series. She earned her MBA (entrepreneurship concentration, perfect GPA) from the Jack Welch Management Institute and built her reputation in corporate sales, entrepreneurship, and strategic consulting.

Bridging science-backed skincare with practical nutrition, Stephanie helps readers transform daily habits into lasting radiance. When she isn't writing or coaching founders, she's developing premium publishing experiences that turn ideas into assets — fast.

Website: www.bookedandbrandedpublishing.com

Series mantra: Glow from the Inside Out.

Made in the USA
Las Vegas, NV
03 November 2026

57420359R00019